Jaqueline Fornari
Carine T. Sangaleti

SALSA and Social Participation Scale

Jaqueline Fornari
Carine T. Sangaleti

SALSA and Social Participation Scale

Perspective of use for nurses' work

ScienciaScripts

Imprint
Any brand names and product names mentioned in this book are subject to trademark, brand or patent protection and are trademarks or registered trademarks of their respective holders. The use of brand names, product names, common names, trade names, product descriptions etc. even without a particular marking in this work is in no way to be construed to mean that such names may be regarded as unrestricted in respect of trademark and brand protection legislation and could thus be used by anyone.

Cover image: www.ingimage.com

This book is a translation from the original published under ISBN 978-613-9-72115-3.

Publisher:
Sciencia Scripts
is a trademark of
Dodo Books Indian Ocean Ltd. and OmniScriptum S.R.L publishing group

120 High Road, East Finchley, London, N2 9ED, United Kingdom
Str. Armeneasca 28/1, office 1, Chisinau MD-2012, Republic of Moldova, Europe
Printed at: see last page
ISBN: 978-620-7-94692-1

I dedicate this work to my mother. For believing that I would be able to get this far and realise this dream.

Thank you

To God for giving me the gift of life and love for the profession I chose to follow.

To my guardian angel who protected me and gave me strength in every difficult moment.

To my parents Mariza Fornari and Aldir Desengrini Fornari, for always giving me strength and believing that I would be able to achieve this dream.

To my dear friend Jessica Thais Bresan for her companionship in difficult and joyful times, for her friendship and loyalty throughout all my years at university.

To my friends Carlos, Leandro, Jonatan, Rodolfo, Eleandro and my friends Bruna and Poliane who have shown their companionship and friendship, providing many moments of joy.

To my teacher and supervisor Carine Teles Sangaleti for her dedication and patience in bringing this work to fruition, and for always sharing her knowledge to help me recognise what to do best and thus do it better and better.

The professors Ms Maria Regiane Trincaus and Ms Maria Luciana, for agreeing to take part in this work and for being admirable people and professionals, I will take a little bit of each one with me. My sincere thanks!

To the patients of the AMPDS for the exchange of experiences, without you this work would not have happened.

Physiotherapist Elisa, who helped me so much and passed on her knowledge so that this work could be carried out.

"Dream and you will be free in spirit... Fight and you'll be free in life"

Ernesto Che Guevara

SUMMARY

FORNARI, Jaqueline. **SALSA and Social Participation Scale: A perspective on its use in nursing work.** 82 pages. Monograph (Graduation) - Department of Nursing. State University of the Centre-West, Guarapuava-PR, 2012.

Leprosy is a chronic infectious disease that is considered a serious public health problem in Brazil, as it is one of the countries with the highest number of cases in the world. It should be noted that the problem of leprosy goes beyond the high number of cases when considering its high disabling potential, as it interferes with the patient's work and social life, as well as causing economic losses and psychological trauma. It is necessary and relevant to find new strategies to improve care for those affected by leprosy. In this context, this study highlights nursing as an area of knowledge capable of working at all levels of care and of structuring itself using various tools to achieve comprehensive care practices for leprosy patients. **Aim:** The aim of this study was to assess the degree of functional activity limitation, risk awareness and social participation of patients after discharge and undergoing treatment for leprosy using the SALSA and Social Participation scales. And based on this evaluation, to promote reflection on the use of these assessments and scales employed in nursing care for leprosy patients at the primary care level. **Population and Methods:** The study population consisted of 30 people undergoing leprosy treatment and post-discharge, all of whom were registered and monitored by the AMPDS in Guarapuava, Paraná. The SALSA and social participation scales were used for data collection, which took place from February to May 2012. The data was analysed and processed using Microsoft Excel 2007 software. **Results:** Of the 30 participants in the study 16 were female and 14 male. With regard to occupation, 40% of the population were on sickness benefit, 33% were retired in most cases due to leprosy, a further 20% had some occupation linked to the informal market with no employment ties and 7% were home workers. Regarding the results of activity limitations, most had some degree of activity limitation. As such: participants with no limitation 3%, mild limitation 38%, moderate limitation 24%, severe limitation 28%, very severe limitation 7%. There was a significant difference in the degree of disability in relation to gender. The degree of risk awareness ranged from 0 to 9. Women scored the highest in terms of risk awareness. With regard to social participation, 73 per cent of people had no significant restriction in social participation. However, 17 per cent had mild restrictions, 7 per cent moderate restrictions and 3 per cent severe restrictions. Women scored higher in social participation restriction than men. **Conclusion:** This research showed that the SALSA and social participation scales can be used in nurses' work, as they were able to provide support for accurate diagnosis and the choice of appropriate nursing interventions for each case, taking into account the complexity of users' health needs. Therefore, these scales are characterised as qualifiers of the nursing care provided to people with or after leprosy discharge.
Key words: 1. leprosy 2. nursing 3. care.

SUMMARY

CHAPTER 1	**6**
CHAPTER 2	**8**
CHAPTER 3	**19**
CHAPTER 4	**24**
CHAPTER 5	**41**
CHAPTER 6	**43**
CHAPTER 7	**48**

CHAPTER 1

INTRODUCTION

Leprosy is a chronic infectious disease caused by a bacillus called Mycobacterium leprae, which is highly infectious and has low pathogenicity. This bacillus mainly affects the integumentary and nervous systems, which is why leprosy manifests itself in skin lesions and neuritic disorders that affect the musculoskeletal system (PEREIRA et al., 2008; BRASIL, 2002). Leprosy is transmitted via the airways through prolonged contact between a susceptible person and a sick person. It is a disease that, if diagnosed and treated early, does not lead to disabilities, deformities and mutilations.

Brazil is one of the countries with the highest number of leprosy cases in the world and the disease is therefore considered a public health problem with an important social dimension. In this context, the most susceptible people belong to unfavourable economic classes, due to the combination of various factors such as the lack of adequate housing conditions, low educational levels and nutritional vulnerabilities (IKEHARA et al., 2010).

It should be emphasised that the problem of leprosy goes beyond the high number of cases when one considers its high disabling potential, as it interferes with the patient's work and social life, as well as causing economic losses and psychological trauma. In addition, these disabilities are responsible for stigma and discrimination against patients (AQUINO et al., 2003). Thus, the damage that leprosy brings to its sufferers is innumerable, and the lack of access and adequate care leads to greater harm.

Based on the above, it is necessary and relevant to find new strategies to improve care for those affected by leprosy. In this context, nursing stands out in this study as an area of knowledge capable of working at all levels of care and of structuring itself using various tools to achieve comprehensive care practices for leprosy patients, since the central axis of its actions is care and not just a limited focus on a pathology or disease. Furthermore, this area of knowledge stands out due to the need for constant renewal according to the needs of the people being cared for.

In the meantime, the Ministry of Health's SALSA (Screening of Activity limitation and Safety Awareness) and social participation scales can be a great ally in identifying the needs of people with leprosy, since they measure activity limitation, risk awareness and restricted social participation in people affected by leprosy (BARBOSA et al., 2008; BRASIL, 2008), thus improving nursing care, with direct intervention in the sequelae left by leprosy.

The main aim of this study was to assess the degree of functional activity limitation, risk awareness and social participation of patients after discharge and undergoing treatment for leprosy using the SALSA and Social Participation scales. And based on this evaluation, to promote reflection on the use of these assessments and scales in nursing care for leprosy patients at primary care level.

CHAPTER 2

THEORETICAL FRAMEWORK

2.1 OVERVIEW OF LEPROSY

Leprosy is a chronic disease characterised as a granulomatous infection caused by the intracellular microorganism Mycobacterium leprae, which was discovered in 1873 by the doctor Amaneur Hansen in Norway. The bacillus has high infective power and low pathogenic power, which is why it requires prolonged contact between the untreated bacilliferous patient and an uncontaminated individual. Leprosy is historically recognised for its incapacitating potential, which is directly related to the bacillus' ability to penetrate nerve cells and cause cell damage, as well as the exacerbated activation of the inflammatory response mediated by the immune system that leads to neuritis. In general, it can be said that the clinical manifestations of leprosy are closely related to the degree of immunity of the person affected, i.e. individual immune characteristics are relevant and explain the different clinical manifestations of leprosy (MENDONÇA et al., 2008; BRASIL, 2002).

Leprosy can take two clinical forms: Paucibacillary, in which the carrier has few bacilli and symptoms characterised by up to five skin lesions; Multibacillary, in which the carrier has many bacilli and more than five skin lesions (WHO, 2006).

According to the WHO (2006) the forms, or clinical classification, are important for determining the treatment that the patient will undergo, which in turn is divided into:

- **Indeterminate leprosy**: initial form, Paucibacillary (PB) characterised by a single lesion or a multiplicity of hypochromic lesions, with imprecise boundaries and decreased or absent sensitivity. In this clinical form, bacilloscopy is negative, i.e. the bacillary load is too low to be identified, but if left untreated it can progress to the other clinical forms of leprosy;
- **Tuberculoid leprosy:** Paucibacillary form, erythematous lesions or plaques with precise boundaries, decreased sensitivity and usually with neurological involvement, presents high specific immunity, i.e. the affected individual has high immunity to the bacillus and will be pointed out with

a negative bacilloscopy;

- **Dimorphic leprosy:** multibacillary (MB) form, lesions characteristic of the tuberculoid and virchowian forms, with erythematous-brownish lesions, plaques, neurological involvement, areas of anaesthesia. Moderate immunity, i.e. the affected individual has immunity to the bacillus but not enough to eliminate it, corresponds to a bacilloscopy with a moderate positive bacillus load;
- **Virvhowian leprosy**: multibacillary form, diffuse infiltration, nodules

disseminated, multiple erythematous-brown lesions, neurological involvement, extensive areas of anaesthesia, low immunity, i.e. the affected individual does not have any immunity against the bacillus, consequently their bacillary load will be very high, showing a strong positive bacillary load on bacilloscopy.

The treatment of leprosy must be immediate in order to prevent nerve damage that can lead to permanent physical disabilities and deformities. This treatment is based on the World Health Organisation's polychemotherapy regimens, which advocated free treatment in endemic countries. In Brazil, it was implemented and standardised in 2001 through the Ministry of Health's ordinance number 1401 (WHO, 2006).

According to the Guide to Leprosy Control, multidrug therapy is appropriate according to the operational classification of leprosy contextualised above:

- Polychemotherapy for paucibacillary forms (MDT - PB): a combination of rifampicin and dapsone is used, with a monthly dose of 600mg of rifampicin (02 capsules of 300mg) + dapsone, a supervised monthly dose of 100mg and a self-administered daily dose. This treatment should last six months. It should be noted that six monthly doses of rifampicin must be supervised. Thus, in the PB forms, discharge is established if the carrier takes the 6 supervised doses within nine months, for the indeterminate and tuberculoid clinical forms,
- Multi-drug therapy for multibacillary forms (MDT-MB): a combination of rifampicin, dapsone and clofazimine, packaged in a tablet, is used as follows: rifampicin: a monthly dose of 600 mg (2 capsules of 300 mg) with supervised administration, clofazimine: a monthly

dose of 300 mg (3 capsules of 100 mg) with supervised administration and a daily dose of 50mg self-administered and dapsone: a monthly dose of 100mg supervised and a daily dose self-administered. In MB forms, the duration of treatment should be 12 months, with 12 supervised monthly doses of rifampicin. The discharge criterion: 12 supervised doses in up to 18 months of treatment (BRASIL, 2002).

Drug treatment is often not a guarantee of freedom from leprosy sequelae, as leprosy reactions, which are acute and sub-acute inflammatory episodes, are one of the main causes of nerve damage and physical disability as a result of the disease, and can occur at the time of leprosy diagnosis, during treatment or after discharge. These reactions are caused by the exacerbation of the patient's immune system's responses to Mycobacterium leprae. Reactive episodes should be treated and do not contraindicate treatment with the standard regimen, which should not be interrupted.

The reactions affecting paucibacillary and multibacillary patients can be of two types:

Type one reaction (I): characterised by worsening of pre-existing lesions, leaving them oedematous, erythematous, shiny and developing into ulcerations. There are also new lesions, infiltration and neuritis.

Type two reaction (II): characterised by erythema nodosum-like lesions, which are erythematous, painful lesions of varying sizes including papules and nodules located anywhere on the skin. In some cases, the reaction may be followed by inflammation of the nerves, joints, iris, testicles and lymph nodes. Reactive hands and feet, proteinuria and liver damage, lower limb oedema and high fever can also occur (ARAUJO, 2003; BRASIL, 2005).

Although there is treatment and a cure for leprosy, its transmission still raises a lot of questions and apprehension among both lay people and health professionals, a fact that reinforces issues of prejudice in relation to this disease. Thus, it must be clear that transmission occurs via the airways, but depends on the prolonged coexistence of susceptible people with a person suffering from MB leprosy who is not undergoing treatment (emphasis added). The onset of the disease in a person infected with the bacillus, and its different clinical manifestations, depend on the parasite/host relationship, among other factors, and can occur after a long incubation period of between two and seven years (BAIALARDI, 2007; BRASIL, 2005).

Leprosy can affect people of all ages and both sexes, however, it rarely occurs in children. It has been observed that children under the age of fifteen fall ill more often when the disease is more endemic. In addition, there is a higher incidence of the disease in men than in women in most regions of the world. In addition to individual conditions, other factors are related to the risk of falling ill, such as: endemic levels of the disease, unfavourable socio-economic conditions with consequent poor living and health conditions and the large number of people living in the same environment (BRASIL, 2002).

In addition to the conditions that favour the risk of falling ill mentioned above, it should be pointed out that the lack of active search for cases or the misguided search for leprosy cases is also a problem for the control and eradication of leprosy. The search for leprosy cases needs to be guided by the evaluation of epidemiological data and the diagnosis is made through anamnesis and dermatoneurological examination, which focuses on investigating neural involvement with thickening of the nerves, accompanied or not by altered sensitivity and/or muscle strength, and especially lesions or areas of the skin with altered sensitivity characterised mainly by whitish or reddish patches, plaque lesions, infiltrations and nodules. A bacilloscopy is the laboratory test that defines the clinical form of leprosy, if it is positive for Mycobacterium leprae (BRASIL, 2005).

In this context, it should be noted that, if diagnosed late, leprosy can cause peripheral neuropathy, which can lead to loss of protective sensitivity, initiated by the infection and accompanied by exacerbation of immunological episodes, whose evolution and sequelae extend for years after the infection is cured. As a result of the neural impairment, there is a loss of protective sensitivity in the hands, feet, eyes and other areas, leading to the appearance of lesions and wounds that can cause functional losses and severe sequelae with consequent physical, psychological and social limitations. It is therefore essential that leprosy is diagnosed early in order to avoid serious complications (BRASIL, 2008a).

2.2 LEPROSY IN BRAZIL: STILL A CHALLENGE

Leprosy continues to be a public health problem in Brazil, as it is one of the countries with the highest number of leprosy cases in the world. Even though it is one of the oldest diseases and the number of cases has been decreasing, 37,610 new cases were registered in 2009 (BRASIL, 2011).

It's worth pointing out that studies indicate that the decrease in the number of cases was due to the introduction of multidrug therapy for the treatment of leprosy, the expansion of the health services that make up the Unified Health System (SUS) and the creation of public policies that provide support for the elimination of leprosy, so it's clear that in order to tackle the problem of leprosy efficiently, it's necessary to work in a network that takes into account various elements of this and not just medication (BRASIL, 2008a; MARTELLI, C.M et al., 2002; CUNHA M.D et al., 2007).

In the North, Midwest and Northeast regions of the country, leprosy case rates are the highest, which is why there is still a need to intensify epidemiological surveillance and leprosy elimination programmes. On the other hand, in regions of Brazil where leprosy is no longer endemic, its diagnostic hypothesis has been disregarded, which leads to late diagnosis of cases and a consequent increase in sequelae and associated disabilities, causing serious damage to the life of the sufferer (SANTOS, 2010; BRASIL, 2006).

In the meantime, Aquino et al. (2003) emphasises that the problem is not just limited to the number of cases, but also to its high incapacitating potential which, if neglected, interferes with the sufferer's work and social life, as well as causing economic losses and psychological trauma. The same author emphasises that disabilities are responsible for stigma and discrimination against sufferers, further damaging their quality of life. The impact of the problem on the public purse also becomes increasingly costly when leprosy cases go unnoticed by health professionals, because when they are diagnosed late, the severity of the disease is already high.

At this point, the strategic role of Primary Care (PC) services in dealing with leprosy should be highlighted, since this level of care should serve as the preferred gateway for SUS users to health services, as well as coordinating the care actions of the other levels in dealing with epidemiological problems of local social relevance. In addition, primary care services are closer to the clientele in each region and can more easily recognise the determinants and conditioning factors of health conditions because they have the potential to use elements that favour active search, longer contact and other aspects as care tools (MOREIRA et al., 2002; FERREIRA et al., 2009; SCHOLZE et.al., 2006; DUARTE; AYRES; SIMONETTI, 2009).

Based on the above, it is necessary for the A B to realise that it plays a fundamental role in tackling leprosy, since many sufferers have had serious sequelae due to late diagnosis. According to the Manual of Disabilities, early diagnosis, the dissemination of information to the population clarifying what leprosy really is, other health education actions, humanised care that encompasses preventive aspects, timely treatment and self-care measures are the main actions for controlling and dealing with leprosy and all these actions should be developed within the scope of primary care (BRASIL, 2008a).

It is essential to maintain effective actions to eliminate leprosy in those regions where the endemic disease has stabilised and to intensify actions in the most endemic areas. However, it should be stressed that all of the above depends on social mobilisation, including the political will of all managers, the commitment and motivation of technicians and the control of civil society (BRASIL, 2008a; LANA F.C.F et al, 2009).

According to the WHO (2006), another challenge in tackling leprosy is the need for a competent referral system that forms part of an integrated information programme, since communication between the participants in this system is fundamental for the proper treatment of a person affected by leprosy or leprosy-related illnesses.

The same author emphasises the need to implement the Operational Guidelines for leprosy control, which in turn were intended to promote the implementation of the Global Strategy for Further Reducing the Leprosy Burden and Sustaining Leprosy Control Activities proposed for 2006-2010.

The expected results at the end of 2010 were a reduction in leprosy levels to very low levels, an increase in the quality of health services with more trained professionals to detect the disease, a better management system, improved quality of case records and accessibility to specialised services; resources to guarantee the prevention of disabilities and rehabilitation when necessary and to promote integration and partnerships with other institutions. (WHO, 2006).

However, the objectives were not met, so in order to reinforce and achieve the objectives of the Global Strategy, the Operational Guidelines were updated and the Enhanced Global Strategy for Further Reducing the Leprosy Burden for the period 2011-2015 was launched, requiring a renewed commitment from all partners working towards the common goal of a world without leprosy (WHO, 2010).

Based on the above, it is understood that the challenge in our country lies in sustaining the quality of leprosy services and ensuring that all people affected by this disease, wherever they live, have an equal opportunity for diagnosis and treatment by competent, committed health professionals, especially those in primary care, through public policies to tackle this social problem, monitoring, eliminating prejudice, disseminating information, training teams in humanised care, and thus maintaining effective work to eliminate leprosy (WHO, 2006; BRAZIL, 2011; BRAZIL, 2008a).

2.3 LEPROSY AND ITS REPERCUSSIONS ON THE LIVES OF SUFFERERS

Due to various causes such as failures in public health, the poor living conditions of a large portion of the Brazilian population, the lack of knowledge about leprosy among health professionals and society in general, stigmas, prejudices and the potential for leprosy to cause physical damage, there are many unfavourable repercussions in the lives of sufferers (AQUINO **et al.,** 2003).

In relation to the body of the person affected by leprosy, what **we call "leprosy implications"** occur, **which are** characterised by dermatoneurological affections, i.e. lesions on the skin and peripheral nerves, mainly in the eyes, hands and feet. These affections cause deformities, spots on the skin, thickening of the nerves, episodes of intense pain during reaction periods, which consequently affect self-image and everyday activities (BRASIL 2008b; MINUZZO, 2008).

And these disabilities that affect many of those affected by leprosy lead to prejudice against the patient by their own family members, who exclude them from socialising, leaving them out of family events, leisure activities and family decision-making, thus making them feel inferior to other people (MARTINS; CAPONI, 2010).

The lack of understanding on the part of leprosy sufferers of the information provided by health professionals, either because it is not given clearly or because they use technical, vague and impersonal language, means that those affected by leprosy seek out other sources of information such as acquaintances, neighbours and relatives, most of whom are laypeople on the subject and therefore pass on incorrect information about the disease. Often, because they don't understand the guidelines, leprosy sufferers isolate themselves and don't share their fears and anxieties, clinging only to their imaginations about the disease. Incorrect or inadequate information not only causes emotional and psychological damage to sufferers, but also increases stigma and prejudice, favouring other people who are not knowledgeable on the subject to exclude the sufferer from community activities, religious festivals, even from greeting the leprosy sufferer with a handshake, for fear of acquiring the disease, as they believe that transmission also occurs through simple contact (NUNES; OLIVEIRA; VIEIRA, 2011; BAIALARDI, 2007).

Another example of discrimination in the lives of leprosy sufferers is from health professionals. Reports from leprosy exporters discuss the role of health professionals in the social institution of prejudice through mistaken measures such as social isolation. In the not so distant past, health professionals were key figures in the institution of stigma against leprosy patients, as they were removed from their families and began to live in an isolated space called colonies, where the patients themselves carried out nursing techniques, without the necessary knowledge or guidance. It should be emphasised that this role performed by the patients themselves was due to a lack of professionals, as they did not accept working with leprosy patients (GUSMÃO; ANTUNES, 2009; MATTOS; FORNAZARI, 2005).

Still in the context of the repercussions on the lives of leprosy sufferers, it should be noted that the population most affected by leprosy is the disadvantaged and economically active class, and that many of those affected by leprosy end up losing their jobs due to the physical limitations caused by the sequelae. In addition, in many cases the affected person is the only source of family income, a fact that makes the family's living conditions even more difficult and consequently jeopardises support for the leprosy sufferer (LANA F.C.F et al.,2009).

In the meantime, even the financial resources earmarked for leprosy patients by the Federal Government have been pointed out as a problem for reinserting patients into the labour market or into a new job, as many of them are unable to find other sources of income besides the benefit, and so they abandon treatment for the sequelae in order to continue receiving sickness benefit (MIRANZI; PEREIRA; NUNES, 2010; BRASIL, 2005). However, it should be emphasised that understanding the problem should not be limited to financial resources, but to the lack of social resources that enable people with the disease to have other perspectives. It is considered that only 1/3 of leprosy sufferers are notified and among these many do not take regular treatment or give up, adding to the impact of the disease (MIRANZI; PEREIRA; NUNES, 2010).

Thus, there are many problems affecting those affected by leprosy, among them prejudice, which is associated with maintaining the stigma that the disease carries.

2.4 NURSING IN THE FIGHT AGAINST LEPROSY

Nursing, which has care as its core competence and responsibility, has the potential to work in different areas of health care, as well as going through the most diverse areas of knowledge to develop care actions, as soon as it is assumed that its focus is on the person being cared for and their needs, and not just the disease. For this reason, nursing can more intensively establish channels of dialogue with agents from other disciplines and, together, seek out the technologies needed for care, establishing relationships with the team and the family, acting in the process of transforming reality (MATUMOTO; MISHIMA; PINTO, 2001). The same authors point out that we should understand nursing today as a practice of relationships, as it always has been and always will be, which uses technological knowledge.

Nursing actions have power as technical-political intervention tools in the health-disease process in order to favour the breaking of causal chains, treatment, rehabilitation and also the prevention of illnesses and health promotion, as well as the control of the healthy (GIROTI; NUNES; RAMOS, 2008). In this context, nursing actions to combat leprosy are supported by the National Leprosy Control Programme (PNCH), which is in line with the SUS principles of access and universality of the right to health, equity and comprehensiveness, respecting the right to citizenship.

It is understood that nursing interventions are a social action and must therefore respond to health needs, which in turn are historically and socially determined (MATUMOTO; MISHIMA; PINTO, 2001). It is therefore possible to think of nursing as an instrument in the fight against leprosy because it has the potential to act as a player in the fight to eliminate it and the stigmas related to it. This aspect is reinforced by the fact that the treatment of leprosy and its aggravating factors requires the articulation of various types of knowledge due to its complex social dimension (IKEHARA et al., 2010).

Nursing care for leprosy patients, especially those diagnosed late in life, requires the use of various tools to achieve effective treatment, and these tools must enable the needs of those who depend on the health service to be identified. It is extremely important to emphasise that the care provided to people affected by leprosy must go beyond the moment of diagnosis and the period of treatment with MDT. The post-discharge period must be considered as relevant from a perspective of longitudinal care and comprehensive care (WHO, 2003).

Based on this contextualisation, leprosy will not cease to be a public health problem if health professionals, especially nurses, maintain a crystallised view only of the disease, failing to take advantage of available resources, or even create and recreate existing ones, with a view to achieving the elimination of leprosy and offering adequate care to users already affected. This emphasises the importance of training nurses to work with leprosy patients, making it essential to use new tools, since they enable a broader view of the health-disease process, facilitating nurses' work with a view to providing comprehensive care (DUARTE; AYRES; SIMONETTI, 2009).

2.5 THE SALSA AND SOCIAL PARTICIPATION SCALES

In view of the above, there are scales designed to identify disabilities, the extent of activity limitation, and to assess awareness of the risks they are exposed to, called the SALSA scale and the social participation assessment scale, which are applicable to leprosy patients and post-discharge patients.

The SALSA (Screening of Activity limitation and Safety Awareness) scale, which in Brazil is translated as Screening of Activity Limitation and Risk Awareness, is a questionnaire made up of twenty items covering four domains: feet, hands and self-care to identify limitations to certain activities due to disabilities caused by leprosy and to assess the risk awareness that the person affected by leprosy has based on carrying out certain activities (BRASIL, 2008a).

The Social Participation Scale is made up of eighteen items and aims to measure perceived problems in the main areas of life such as learning and applying knowledge; communication and personal care; mobility; domestic life; interpersonal and community interactions. This scale uses the concept of PAR, i.e. comparison between similar individuals. Despite being a term that is still little known and used by the general population, the concept of PAR aims to eliminate differences in participation resulting from gender and social class (BRASIL, 2008a).

The use of these scales is still limited in the daily practice of health services, but according to studies that have evaluated their applicability, the SALSA and Social Participation scales can favour the diagnosis of specific needs in the context of leprosy (IKEHARA et al., 2010).

CHAPTER 3

CASUISTRY AND METHOD

3.1 TYPE OF STUDY

This was a descriptive, cross-sectional quantitative study carried out at the Municipal Pneumology and Health Dermatology Outpatient Clinic (AMPDS) in the municipality of Guarapuava, PR.

The main objective of descriptive research is to describe the characteristics of a particular population or phenomenon (GIL, 2006). The cross-sectional study involves collecting data at a point in time, from which the phenomena under study are reached during a period of data collection (BONITA, 2010).

3.2 STUDY SITE

The study was carried out on the premises of the Municipal Pneumology and Dermatology Outpatient Clinic (AMPDS) in the municipality of Guarapuava, PR, which serves as a reference centre for the treatment of respiratory diseases, primarily tuberculosis, and dermatological diseases, especially leprosy. The AMPDS carries out the decentralisation policy of the National Leprosy Control Programme.

Leprosy (PNCH) with supervision, in-service training and monitoring of leprosy care in the basic health network of that municipality and referrals for medium-complexity care to municipalities belonging to the 5ª Regional Health Centre.

3.3 STUDY POPULATION

The study population was made up of 30 people who had been affected by leprosy or were undergoing treatment for the disease, who were registered and being monitored by the AMPDS team in Guarapuava, PR, during the months of February to May 2012 (data collection period).

The inclusion criteria for this study were: being a leprosy patient undergoing treatment or a post-discharge user, being registered and actively followed up at the Guarapuava Municipal Pneumology and Dermatology Outpatient Clinic, living in the municipality of Guarapuava-PR and having the availability and cognitive conditions to answer the SALSA and Social Participation scales during the period stipulated for data collection in this study.

3.4 DATA COLLECTION

Data collection took place between February and May 2012. Copies of the Ministry of Health's SALSA and Social Participation scales were used.

The SALSA scale (Appendix 01) aims to measure the extent of activity limitation and the awareness of risk to factors that can increase impairments when carrying out activities. It was developed to be applied to those affected by leprosy, diabetes mellitus or other peripheral neuropathies. The SALSA scale covers four types of domains involving hands, feet and self-care, so it serves to identify limitations for certain activities resulting from disabilities caused by leprosy, as well as assessing the risk awareness that the person affected by leprosy has about carrying out certain activities which, if poorly performed, can aggravate the degree of physical impairment (BRASIL, 2008a).

The Social Participation Scale (Annex 02) measures the degree of severity of restriction of the social activities of those affected by leprosy. **It uses the "PAR" concept which, despite being a term little known and** used by the general population, is intended to eliminate differences in perception of the degree of social participation resulting from gender and social class. The PAR concept is used as follows: the interviewee is asked to think of a person who is almost the same age as them, who has the same social class conditions, whether or not they are related to the interviewee, but who has <u>not</u> been affected by leprosy. After thinking about this element (the PAR individual), the person with leprosy is asked about situations involving social participation, asking them to compare themselves with the PAR. In this way, it is possible to get a sense of how much leprosy has affected their social life compared to a similar individual who has not had the disease (BRASIL, 2008a).

3.2.1 Data Collection Procedure

In order to apply the scales, the availability of a room within the AMPDS for the interview was requested. The interviewees were all people affected by leprosy who were in treatment or post-discharge from the disease, and the interviews were scheduled by the outpatient physiotherapist according to the availability of each participant.

In order to favour the participation of the research subjects and the field researcher's ability to use the SALSA and Social Participation scales, a voluntary internship was carried out at the AMPDS for one year and six months prior to the collection period. During this internship, care activities were carried out with leprosy patients and with those who had already been discharged but were still being monitored in the service due to sequelae.

The internship took place between December 2010 and May 2012. Through these activities, a bond was established with the users, reducing their discomfort at taking part in a survey that used a scale to collect data.

Also in this context, it should be noted that there was already an established partnership between the proponents of this study.

The scales were applied in accordance with the instructions recommended by the Ministry of Health in the Disability Prevention Manual number 1. Once the scales had been applied, the data was tabulated and then analysed.

3.4.2Definition of variables and their indicators

In this study, the variables investigated were: gender, age, schooling, occupation, activity limitations, risk awareness and social participation. Below is a description of each variable.

Sex: Variable categorised into two groups: Male; Female.

Age: Numeric variable collected in years of age.

Occupation: Variable categorised into four groups: Working; Retired; Sickness benefit; Household.

Activity limitation: The SALSA scale (ANNEX 01) covers five domains involving eyes, hands (dexterity and work), feet (mobility) and self-care. The score ranges from 10 to 80. The lower the score, the less difficulty with activities of daily living and higher scores indicate increasing levels of activity limitation.

activities (BRASIL, 2008a).

This variable was categorised into five groups, as indicated on the SALSA scale itself: Ten to twenty-four (no limitation); Twenty-five to thirty-nine (mild limitation); Forty to forty-nine (moderate limitation); Fifty to fifty-nine (severe limitation); Sixty to eighty (very severe limitation).

Risk awareness: The second score is the risk awareness score. During the interview, the interviewer must tick one answer option for each of the questions asked. To calculate the safety awareness score, count the number of options that have a four with a circle around them. The result is a score between zero and eleven. Higher scores indicate a growing awareness of the risks involved in certain activities, but also indicate that there is a limitation of activity as a result (BRASIL, 2008a).

Social participation: The score on the Social Participation Scale (ANNEX 02) ranges from zero to ninety points. The degrees of restriction were classified as follows: Zero to twelve (no significant restriction); Thirteen to twenty-two (slight restriction); Twenty-three to thirty-two (moderate restriction); Thirty-three to fifty-two (severe restriction); Fifty-three to ninety (extreme restriction) (BRASIL, 2008a).

3.5 ANALYSING THE DATA

The data obtained was initially collected on paper questionnaires and then tabulated and processed using Microsoft Excel 2007 software. Descriptive statistics were carried out on the variables, which were stratified by gender, using mean and standard deviation for numerical variables and prevalence for categorical variables. Descriptive statistics were also carried out using Microsoft Excel 2007 software.

3.6 ETHICAL ASPECTS

All the individuals who took part in the research signed an informed consent form.

The research project was registered with the National Information System on Ethics in Research Involving Human Beings, in accordance with the norms of Resolution 196/96 of the National Health Council. This project was also assessed and authorised by the Research Ethics Committee of the Midwestern State University (COMEP/UNICENTRO), opinion no. 259/2011.

All the individuals who took part in the research signed an informed consent form.

CHAPTER 4

RESULTS AND DISCUSSIONS

The items below present the results of parameters related to leprosy patients and post-discharge users interviewed at the Municipal Dermatology and Pneumology Outpatient Clinic in Guarapuava, Paraná.

4.1 GENDER, AGE AND OCCUPATION.

In this study, 30 people affected by leprosy were interviewed, of whom 16 were female (53.3%) and 14 were male (46.7%). As for gender, there was no significant difference in the proportion of men and women, while the literature shows that the predominance of those affected by leprosy is male (BRASIL, 2002; BRASIL, 2006; GOMES et al., 2005; MIRANZI; PEREIRA; NUNES, 2010; DINIZ et al., 2009).

Rather than being a gender issue, it is possible that the higher prevalence among men is due to the profile of occupational activities that they carry out to a greater extent (MARCKERT, 2008). In addition to the occupational aspects, Melão et al. (2011) point out that the prevalence among men is also due to the broader nature of social interaction, as well as less concern for the body and care for the body.

own health among them.

The population interviewed ranged in age from 35 to 78, with an average age of 55.5. Graph 1 shows that the prevalent age group was 44-54 years old, so they were in the economically active age group. This is in line with the literature, which emphasises that leprosy is prevalent in the economically active (GOMES. et al., 2005; MIRANZI; PEREIRA; NUNES, 2010; DINIZ et al., 2009; BARBOSA et al., 2008).

This finding, in line with many other studies, shows that factors outside the home are more relevant to leprosy infection. At this point, we must emphasise that it is common for health workers and society in general to stick to control and/or other types of interventions focused on the homes of leprosy patients, such as hygiene conditions, contact with communicants and so on. The prevalence rate of leprosy in the adult and economically active age group shows that control and care actions must seek out other sources of contagion and dissemination that have perpetuated the disease in the country.

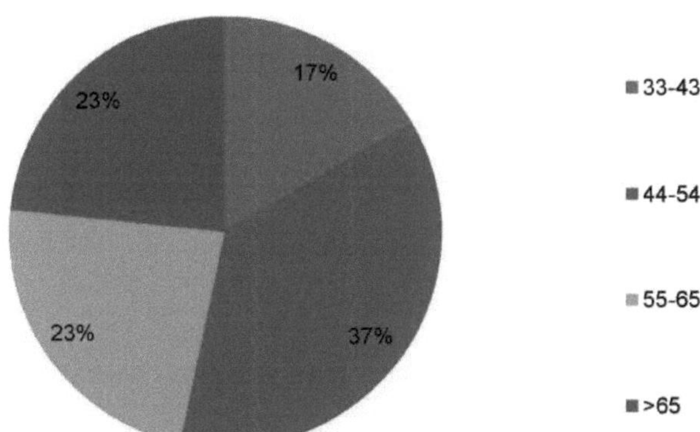

Graph 1- Percentage distribution according to age group of post-discharge and leprosy treatment patients at the Municipal Dermatology Pneumology Outpatient Clinic, Guarapuava, PR, 2012.

SOURCE: THE AUTHOR

Another relevant fact shown in Graph 1 is the lower prevalence of leprosy among younger people. Historically, epidemiological data has shown that leprosy is rare in children, adolescents and the younger age group. Cases of leprosy in these age groups occur in situations of intense endemicity, so they portray alarming situations; this is not the case in the municipality studied. This data also strengthens the argument about the sources of infection and spread of leprosy being related to occupational issues outside the home. However, the occurrence of leprosy cases in children in Brazil can still be considered an indicator of the prevalence of the disease, in other words, it is an indicator that shows that the goals of eliminating the disease have not been achieved. In Brazil, the state with the highest endemic rate of leprosy in children is Amazonas (IMBIRIBA. et al., 2008).

In this context, the state of Paraná has the highest number of leprosy cases in the southern region, and is the only state in this region where leprosy is still endemic. With regard to the prevalence rate in children, the rates of 1.13 and 1.22 cases per 10,000 inhabitants in the Cianorte and Ivaiporã Health Regions in 2005 were hyperendemic, according to Ministry of Health parameters. And in the regions of Guarapuava and Cascavel, with a coefficient of 0.40 cases per 10,000 inhabitants, also in 2005, among children under 15, these regions were considered to be highly endemic (SOBRINHO; MATHIAS, 2008).

Still on the subject of prevalence rates found in epidemiological studies based on secondary data, it is important to reflect on the veracity of zero or low numbers of leprosy cases in various regions of the state of Paraná and even in other Brazilian states where the human development index, working conditions and income, among other parameters that favour the occurrence of leprosy are present. It should be noted here that the municipality in question, Guarapuava, has a well-defined leprosy control and treatment programme run by the AMPDS team, which coordinates the work carried out throughout the basic network. Thus, a low incidence is not a reason to be unconcerned, but rather to mobilise professionals with radio and newspaper campaigns, meetings with UBS teams and active case search campaigns (PONTES, 2010).

Ocupação

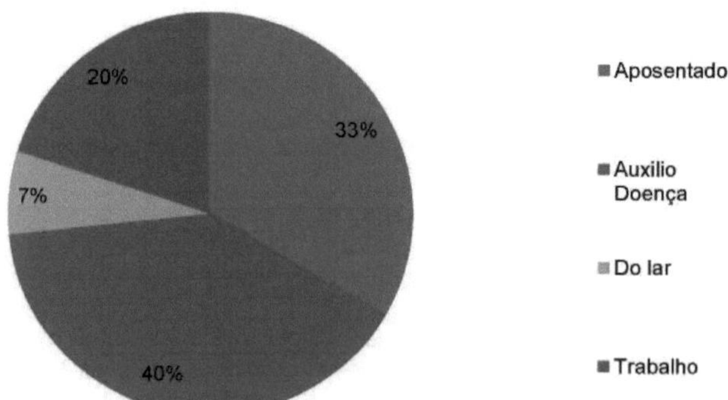

Graph 2- Percentage distribution according to occupation of post-discharge and leprosy treatment patients at the Municipal Dermatology Pneumology Outpatient Clinic, Guarapuava, PR, 2012

SOURCE: THE AUTHOR

Labour* = not employed and linked to the informal labour market.

With regard to the occupation of those interviewed, as shown in Graph 2, the majority are in the productive labour force, which reflects the population base from which the population affected by leprosy in Guarapuava comes. In this context, in a study carried out in 2002, Helene and Salum (2002) showed that leprosy is a health problem that reflects the social reproduction of precarious living and working conditions. This study, like Ribeiro Júnior, Vieira and Caldeira (2012), shows that this consideration can still be taken as contemporary, since leprosy is a disease that affects poor people belonging to socially excluded classes.

As shown in Graph 2, most of the patients interviewed are retired or receive sickness benefit. This predominant condition may be associated with the incapacitating power of leprosy.

In this context, Aquino et al. (2003) state that the problem of leprosy is not just limited to the number of cases (the prevalence), but also to the high incapacitating power which, if neglected, interferes with the work and social life of the sufferer, as well as causing economic losses. In this context, the study by Silva Sobrinho and Mathias (2008) helps to clarify this high rate of absence from work, as it shows that leprosy is diagnosed late in the state of Paraná, especially the multibacillary forms, such as Virchovian leprosy, which has a high incapacitating power.

The study in question also emphasises that low prevalence rates of the disease, as is the case in the states of Santa Catarina and Rio Grande do Sul, do not necessarily represent the elimination of cases, but may represent negligence on the part of the health sector and malpractice on the part of professionals in diagnosing or even having leprosy as a diagnostic hypothesis.

In these two states, for example, there are few cases, but they are identified in very advanced stages of the disease, with consequent disabling repercussions for sufferers (MELÃO et al., 2011).

It is also worth pointing out that financial aid for leprosy sufferers is often seen as a problem in terms of reintegrating them into the labour market or finding a new job, as many of them abandon treatment for the sequelae in order to continue receiving sickness benefit (MIRANZI; PEREIRA;

NUNES, 2010). This factor demonstrates the fragility of the health system and other social support networks, whose inefficiency favours abandoning treatment in order to maintain resources. A study by Luna et al. (2010) of leprosy patients with limited work activities and patients undergoing treatment without sequelae showed that work is the main daily activity among patients, and that leaving work is identified as a factor that distorts their social identity and thus perpetuates patterns of exclusion, lack of adherence, lack of self-care and difficulty in reintegrating into more organised patterns of life.

Leprosy-related absence from work is directly related to the onset of disabilities that result in limited functional activities. Therefore, the data in this study shows the magnitude of the sequelae resulting from this disease. In this context, there is no need to pass judgement on leprosy sufferers who abandon treatment in order to maintain financial support, but there is a need to implement health and social security policies capable of preventing sequelae and guaranteeing the reintegration of individuals into appropriate work activities, under conditions of sequelae. Dias and Pedrazzani (2008) showed that the effective and monitored implementation of actions to prevent disabilities in the basic health network was able to significantly reduce the onset of disabilities and, with these actions, reduce the degree of social exclusion of people with leprosy.

4.2 ACTIVITY LIMITATION

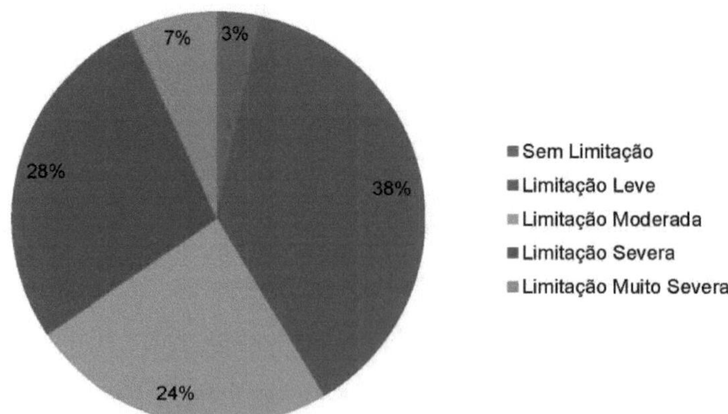

Graph 3- Percentage distribution of activity limitation of post-discharge and leprosy treatment patients at the Municipal

Dermatology Pneumology Outpatient Clinic, Guarapuava, PR, 2012 SOURCE: THE AUTHOR

Supporting the discussion on occupation, graph 3 shows that most of the interviewees had some degree of activity limitation, which may be associated with the unfavourable repercussions that leprosy has on patients. This data also reinforces the argument about the late diagnosis of incapacitating multibacillary forms highlighted by Sobrinho and Mathias (2008) in the state of Paraná.

Studies show that the majority of leprosy sufferers have some degree of physical impairment as a result of the disease. The determinants of these repercussions are not only the disease itself, but also the timing of the diagnosis, which in many cases happens late, as mentioned above. In this context, it is worth emphasising again that in regions where leprosy is not endemic, leprosy cases go unnoticed by health professionals, and when they are diagnosed, the disease is at a very advanced stage, causing an increase in sequelae and associated disabilities (SANTOS, 2010; BRASIL, 2006).

Although the diagnosis is simple, clinical in most cases, many professionals find it difficult to recognise leprosy (ARANTES et al., 2010). Therefore, professional unpreparedness is also a factor in the perpetuation of leprosy in Brazil.

In addition to poor diagnosis, care that is limited to drug treatment and does not take into account the living conditions of the patient, the degree to which the patient understands how to receive information can favour the onset of disabilities (BAIALARDI, 2007). Lack of access to health services and inadequate living conditions also favour negative repercussions (AQUINO et al., 2003 ; ALVES et al., 2010; SOBRINHO et.al, 2007).

4.3 ACTIVITY LIMITATION X GENDER

It was considered relevant in this study to broaden our understanding of gender issues related to leprosy, considering that these issues permeate the vast majority of health problems and social support in our country.

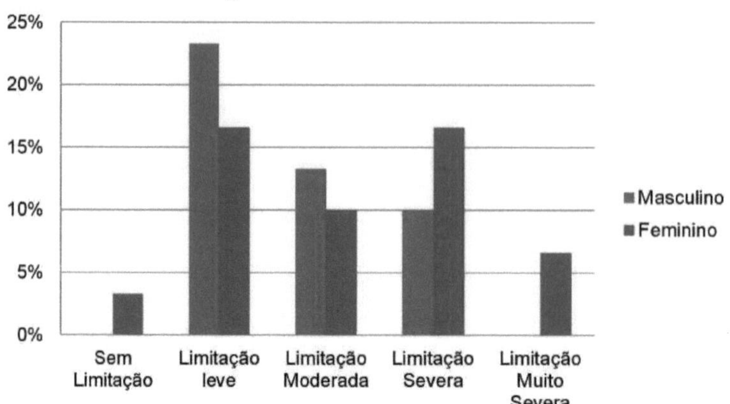

Graph 4- Percentage distribution of activity limitation comparing the sex of post-discharge and leprosy treatment patients at the Municipal Dermatology Pneumology Outpatient Clinic, Guarapuava, PR, 2012.

SOURCE: THE AUTHOR

Graph 4 shows that there are differences in the degree of disability according to gender. In the comparative relationship between activity limitation and gender, women have the highest degrees of activity limitation. Thus, the data from this study contradicts the vast majority of national studies, such as those by Lana et al (2008), which show that men are at greater risk and have a higher rate of physical activity limitation as a result of leprosy sequelae.

Leprosy is a disease in which a possible and common sequel is neural insensitivity to pain, touch or any other type of contact with the hands and feet. As the onset of the disease occurs mostly in adulthood, a period in which we have established behavioural habits, handling kitchen utensils, washing clothes and other household chores do not take into account the care needed to avoid major leprosy sequelae such as burns, wounds, clawed hands and feet, atrophy and many others that lead to limited activity.

However, in the social context of the activities attributed to women, it is certain that they tend to be overburdened to carry out their domestic chores, as well as facing the care required for leprosy treatment (OLIVEIRA; ROMANELLI, 1998). In the meantime, the often triple working day is characterised as an aggravating factor or potential for injuries and consequent disabilities in women's lives.

Despite the fact that women have historically been recognised as better carers, in situations where habits are incorporated, especially those related to the domestic environment, women's vulnerability to developing sequelae increases.

Still from a gender perspective, the impact of limited functional activity on women's lives must be considered. In other diseases such as myocardial infarction, breast cancer and bowel cancer in which functional activity limitation occurs, studies show that the repercussions of these are different in women when compared to men who have had their activity limited by the same or similar limiting illnesses, which are generally worse in women (LEMOS, et al., 2008; FAVARATO , et al., 2006).

Thus, it is not uncommon for women with limited functional activities to suffer from depression, anxiety, self-esteem deficits and to be even less recognised and valued in their own family or personal networks, so the gender difference related to functional limitations is another factor to be considered in leprosy care (LEMOS, et al., 2008; FAVARATO , et al., 2006).

4.3 RISK AWARENESS

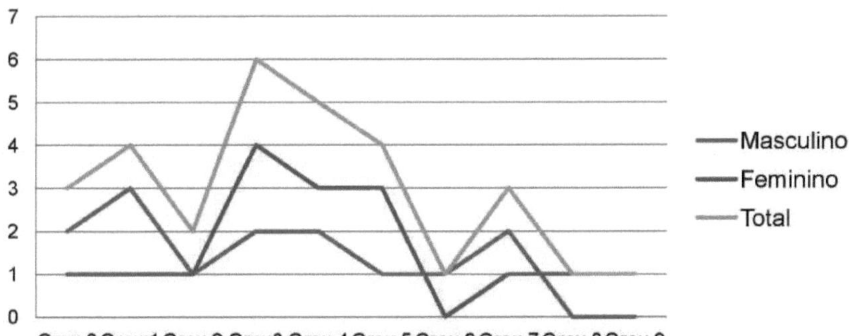

Graph 5 - Frequency distribution of the degree of risk awareness regarding the performance of activities by post-discharge and leprosy treatment patients at the Municipal Dermatology Pneumology Outpatient Clinic, Guarapuava, PR, 2012.

SOURCE: THE AUTHOR

As shown in graph 5, the degree of risk awareness of the participants in this study ranged from 0 to 9. As emphasised in this paper, higher scores indicate increasing degrees of risk awareness involved in certain activities, but also indicate that there is a limitation of activity as a result (BRASIL, 2008a).

The degree of awareness reflects the quality of care the patient is receiving, since they have the limitation, but are aware of the risk of carrying out certain activities that could increase the risk of sequelae.

On the other hand, when those affected by leprosy have low levels of risk awareness, this shows us just how much people with leprosy are aware of the risk.

sequelae are likely to cause greater damage to themselves, since physical sequelae profoundly alter the patient's life condition and when not properly cared for can increase the degree of complexity/impact of the disease, such as evolving with physical alterations that change appearance and cause severe physical limitations in the performance of daily activities (BARBOSA et al., 2008; BRASIL, 2008b).

The degree of risk awareness can and should be related to the degree of understanding, schooling and cultural differences of those affected by leprosy, because if these aspects are disregarded at the time of guidance, the information is invalid, not because the person is uninterested in taking care of themselves, but because the information is not understood.

It is worth emphasising once again that the patient's living conditions, the possibilities of caring for themselves and the quality of the health services on offer are closely linked to the promotion of self-care for those affected by leprosy (BRASIL, 2002; AQUINO et al., 2003; LUNA. I.T et al., 2010).

Although the female participants in this study had higher levels of activity limitation, on the other hand they scored the highest levels of risk awareness, which is in line with what Brasil (2008) points out that higher risk awareness scores also indicate that there is an activity limitation, and this limitation implies having to be more attentive to risk issues. This data implies an enquiry into the degree of functional limitation of the study population at the time of diagnosis in the health services, so that arguments can be inferred in more depth about the ways of looking after one's own health, the degree of body perception and other parameters related to the indicators of the degree of activity limitation and awareness of risk in terms of gender. No study was found that made such a correlation.

Perhaps the historical characteristic of women in taking care of themselves prevails after they acquire activity limitations, even in situations of long-acquired household habits; or women adhere more to the guidance they receive in health services, or health professionals, because they are mostly women, perform better in guidance with women, as studies on men's health in Brazil point out (COUTO et al., 2010; FIGUEIREDO, 2005).

This study also compared the degree of activity limitation with the level of risk awareness, as this data should be used in this way. The lower the level of risk awareness, the greater the risk of loss of functional activity, even in situations where there is no disability or loss of activity. What's more, the higher the degree of risk awareness, the better the health care actions offered in a service. Therefore, this comparative data serves to monitor the care provided to leprosy patients, as well as monitoring the health service itself.

Table 01- Comparison of the classification of Activity limitation with the result of the Degree of Risk Awareness, of post-discharge and leprosy treatment patients at the Municipal Dermatology Pneumology Outpatient Clinic, Guarapuava, PR, 2012.

Activity Limitation	**NO**	**Percentage**	**Risk Awareness**
No Limitation	1	3,3%	0
Slight limitation	12	40%	0 a 3
Moderate Limitation	7	23,3%	2 a 5
Severe Limitation	8	26,6%	5 a 8
Very Severe Limitation	2	6,6%	7 a 9
Total	**30**		

It is interesting to note that, as shown in the table above, the greater the limitation, the greater the risk awareness in the population studied. This shows that although patients have limitations, they are aware of the risks.

As previously pointed out, high levels of activity limitation are related to late diagnosis, lack of access to health services, unqualified staff and precarious living conditions. On the other hand, high levels of risk awareness show that the care provided has taken into account the daily aspects of this population's life. Another factor that reinforces this argument was the fact that the population studied was regularly monitored and integrated with the AMPDS team. This was made possible by a long-term internship at the site and previous contact with the population studied, as presented in the methodological section of this study.

It is worth noting that this result may reflect the quality of care provided to leprosy patients during the course of their treatment, since despite the limitation of functional activity, the degrees of risk awareness are high in the most compromised cases, which demonstrates the user's understanding of the disease that affects or has affected them, It also favours quality of life parameters such as the empowerment of people affected by leprosy, encouraging them to play an active role in their rehabilitation process (BRASIL, 2008a).

If the degrees of activity limitation are directly related to the time of diagnosis and the quality of care during treatment, it is possible for patients or former patients to have their condition alleviated or functional impairment avoided if diagnosis is rapid and care is qualified.

On the other hand, the scores obtained in this study show that those with mild limitations or no limitations have low levels of risk awareness, probably due to the degree of limitation itself, which should also be noted (BRASIL, 2008a).

4.4 SOCIAL PARTICIPATION

Leprosy is one of the diseases or health problems that still arouses a lot of prejudice today, as it is loaded with stigmas. For this reason, verifying the levels or perceptions of patterns of social participation among those who have or have had leprosy is fundamental to tackling the problem in question. Despite this, studies on this issue are very scarce.

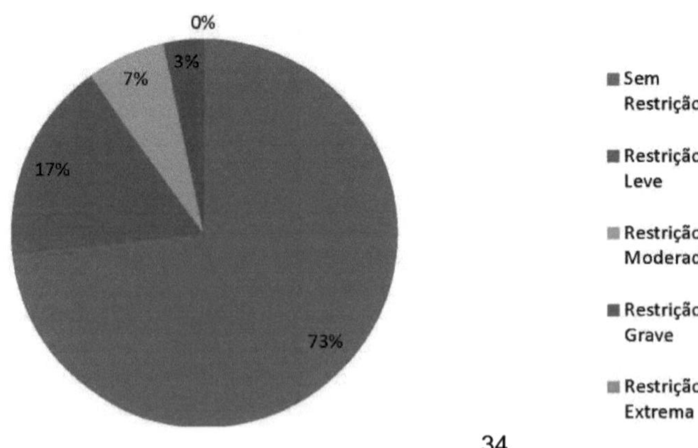

Graph 6 - Percentage distribution of the degree of social participation of post-discharge and leprosy treatment patients at the Municipal Dermatology Pneumology Outpatient Clinic, Guarapuava, PR, 2012.

SOURCE: THE AUTHOR

Analysing Graph 6, with the percentages obtained from the Social Participation Scale, shows that the majority of people had no significant restrictions on their social participation.

All the participants in this study who have no restriction in social participation, when related to activity limitation data, ranged from no limitation to moderate limitation.

The correlation between the SALSA risk perception score and the Participation Scale classification showed that all the participants classified as having no restriction in social participation were distributed across practically all the SALSA scale scores. As discussed elsewhere, the relationship between gender and levels of restricted social participation was investigated. Again, there were differences between the sexes, with possible gender implications.

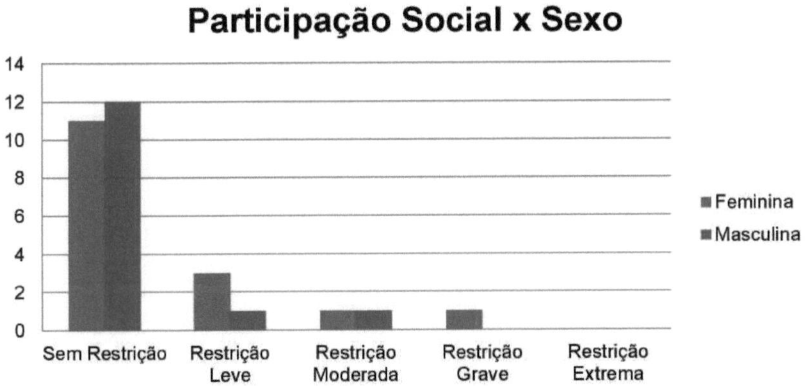

Participação Social x Sexo

14
12
10
8
6
4
2
0
Sem Restrição
Restrição Leve
Restrição Moderada
Restrição Grave
Restrição Extrema
Feminina
Masculina

Graph 7 - Frequency distribution of the degree of social participation by gender of patients after discharge and undergoing treatment for leprosy at the Municipal Dermatology Pneumology Outpatient Clinic, Guarapuava, PR, 2012.

SOURCE: THE AUTHOR

Graph 7 shows that when we relate the social participation data to the gender of the study participants, among the 23 participants classified as having no significant restrictions, 12 (52.17%) are male and 11 (47.83%) are female. Analysing the correlation between a specific gender and the degree of social participation showed that women have higher degrees of social participation restriction than men.

Once again, the data in this study points to gender-related issues, with a disadvantage for women. This may be related to the degree of activity limitation, which is greater among women, or to the implications of these functional limitations in the context of women's lives, as discussed above. A study reveals that in terms of health, women and men show significant differences, not only in terms of specific needs, but also in terms of access to health protection. It is known that the disease can be a trigger for changes in family structure, putting women affected by leprosy at a disadvantage due to the double discrimination they suffer, i.e. they are discriminated against on the basis of their gender and the fact that they are ill (OLIVEIRA; RAMANELLI, 1998).

Table 02 - Characteristics of patients with restricted social participation, post-discharge and undergoing leprosy treatment at the Municipal Dermatology Pneumology Outpatient Clinic, Guarapuava, PR, 2012.

N0	Age	Sex	EP	Limiting activity
1	56	M	MR	LL
2	55	M	LR	LS
3	39	F	LR	LM
4	54	F	GR	LS
5	62	F	LR	LMS
6	70	F	LR	LS
7	53	F	MR	LMS
Total	7			

Note: EP- Participation Scale Classification, MR- Moderate Restriction, LR- Slight Restriction, GR- Severe Restriction, LL- Slight Limitation, LS- Severe Limitation, LMS- Very Severe Limitation.

Analysing table 02, it can be seen that all the patients with restricted participation have some degree of activity limitation. Patients with restricted social participation totalled 7 patients (23.3%) of the total sample. There was a predominance of 5 females (71.42%) and 2 males (28.57%). Their ages ranged from 39 to 70. Regarding the degree of social participation, it should be noted that despite the stigmatising nature of leprosy, limitation of activities was more present than restriction of social participation in all degrees of disability and did not always correlate.

Most of the participants in this study had no restrictions on their social participation, as found in the few studies that have used the Social Participation Scale in Brazil (BARBOSA et al., 2008) and unlike the studies on the impact of prejudice on the social relationships of leprosy patients (NUNES; OLIVEIRA; VIEIRA , 2011; BAIALARDI, 2007).

Thus, except for the condition of reintegration into the labour market, the data from this study shows that leprosy in the population studied has been tackled efficiently to break down prejudices and allow social coexistence among peers. We can once again associate this rate with the attention received in the health network, more specifically in the AMPDS and basic health units in Guarapuava (PONTES, 2010). In addition, SUS initiatives via the media and educational and screening campaigns have been supporting the elimination of leprosy and the dissemination of real information in society (WHO, 2006; MARTELLI et al., 2002; CUNHA et al., 2007).

4.6 SALSA AND SOCIAL PARTICIPATION SCALE: PERSPECTIVES FOR USE AS A TOOL IN NURSING CARE: WEAKNESSES AND POTENTIALITIES

The data obtained using the SALSA and Social Participation Scales imply a series of actions in the sphere of health services, social security and society in general in relation to leprosy. This study, however, focuses on nursing as an area of knowledge present at all levels of care within the SUS, especially at primary level, where it has stood out since the first Brazilian initiatives to reinvert healthcare models.

It is common for nurses to qualify their care actions by applying scales in the most diverse lines of work, such as oncology, children's health, workers' health, patients with chronic diseases, ulcers and many others. The use of these instruments, however, should be seen as a stage in their work process and not limited to obtaining a parameter of purely bureaucratic value, as is often the case in the same lines of work mentioned above.

The application of the scales showed that they can serve as instruments in nursing care for leprosy patients, since their purpose is to identify the impact that leprosy has had on the lives of patients, both in their biological bodies and in their social lives, so that a broader view can be obtained of the damage that leprosy has brought to the lives of each patient, for later intervention. Potentiating the focus of nursing care that goes beyond curative practice.

It is of great value to point out that these instruments help to organise the health service, since the actions provided to leprosy patients can be planned according to each need and thus offer a higher quality of care.

In this context, the SALSA scale, which describes the risk awareness that a person affected by leprosy has about carrying out daily activities, can then be used to prevent sequelae based on the patient's own circumscribed perception and not just that of the nurse. The SALSA scale also reflects the pattern of self-care, which is a dimension that is often addressed in nurses' care actions.

As pointed out in this study, nurses can also use the SALSA scale to assess the care provided to leprosy patients, as it is hoped that the disease is diagnosed early so that the sequelae that limit activity have not set in, and that during treatment the level of risk awareness increases and limitations do not occur or do not evolve, if the patient is diagnosed with limitations in place.

A more complex aspect that requires more attention from nurses is gender-related issues. It is said that the object of the work is not limited to the disease, but includes social and cultural aspects, among others. Therefore, gender issues closely related to the cultural and social context must be taken into account in the results obtained from the use of scales. The results of the SALSA scale showed that it is not enough to analyse the scores obtained by the scale individually, but that it is also necessary to carry out a comparative study of all the service users. And this study has shown that this assessment is valid not only in the presence of leprosy, but also among former leprosy sufferers, who often have sequelae or still have a certain stigma about the disease.

Some of the interviewees were identified as having leprosy sequelae, such as loss of protective sensitivity in their hands. Because they had burns, they said they didn't know how they got them, but at the end of applying the scale they realised that they had grade 1 risk awareness, so they didn't realise that they were caused by certain activities carried out without protection. The nursing intervention was to provide guidance and show how these activities can be carried out with adaptations to avoid certain damage to them.

The needs of people with disabilities can be understood through interventions that are specific to each individual and their family members, and that consider the communities in which they live. Interventions that benefit the whole community, directly or indirectly, will further develop community participation and ownership.

In the meantime, the Ministry of Health's Social Participation scale serves as a nursing care tool for people affected by leprosy. Its questions aim to identify patterns of exclusion in the family, community and society in general.

The results obtained in this study using this scale show the relevance of the possible impacts of appropriate health care actions. Therefore, by using this scale, nurses can broaden their focus on the real focal points of exclusion, such as family, community, work and even health services, with a view to reducing social stigmas that can have more severe repercussions than the loss of bodily functionality itself.

It was identified that the professional-patient bond, and in the case of this study, researcher-user, favours the use of instruments, as the answers obtained are easily presented with the user's interest. The results obtained in this study subsidised the creation of a group with users that discusses self-care actions in the AMPDS to share doubts and guidance on caring for activities of daily living that can cause sequelae. This action demonstrates professional commitment to users, and so the use of scales is no longer carried out solely with the focus on the bureaucracy of monthly care.

On the other hand, the absence of professional commitment, lack of interest or effort to adapt the forms of communication with users with or former patients with leprosy can lead to mistrust and lack of adherence due to misunderstanding of the care plan or simply the guidance given.

A calm, quiet environment that provides privacy favours the application of the scale, as the patient feels safe answering the questions. Adequate language is essential, and this requires an interest in getting to know the patient, showing interest in the answers and their importance for improving their state of health. However, it is essential to make it clear at this point that clarity of language cannot change the meaning of the questions in the scales.

The bond that the patients had with the health service where the study took place and the team in question collaborated positively, since they showed tranquillity and security in answering the questions. It is also important to emphasise that the solutions to the problems that appeared according to the data obtained on the scale were explained and discussed with the patient with a view to finding the best solutions.

CHAPTER 5

CONCLUSION

The survey made it possible to gauge the degree to which participants were limited in their activities: the majority of those interviewed had some degree of limitation and when this data was related to gender, women had a higher degree of activity limitation; despite this, women also had a higher degree of risk awareness when carrying out activities of daily living. With regard to Social Participation, the majority of interviewees had no restrictions.

It was found that the SALSA and Social Participation scales can be used in everyday primary care services, and especially in the work of nurses, as they were able to provide support for a more accurate diagnosis and the choice of appropriate nursing interventions for each case. This is an innovative aspect of this research, as there are no studies from this perspective in Brazil in the field of primary care.

The focus of this study is that the SALSA and Social Participation Scales are elements that qualify nurses' care actions and can even guide the process of systematising care in the primary health care setting.

It is worth emphasising that the results of the scales express the perception that the user himself, in this case a leprosy carrier or former carrier, has of his limitations, risk awareness and social participation, and are not limited to the conceptions that professionals have of him, which contributes to adherence to the health professional's conduct.

The results obtained through the scales showed that leprosy interferes with the ability of affected individuals to carry out their daily activities, regardless of the limitations they have, but interventions/adaptations can be made so that activities can be carried out without potentiating the damage caused by leprosy in the lives of those affected by it.

Based on the data presented, it is possible to understand that health work must challenge the simplicity of numerical scores and consider the complexity of the health problems that are often translated into these scores. This became clear when considering the gender issues identified.

In this context, the SALSA and Social Participation scales can be used by nursing professionals in their work process to identify and highlight problems. It is a complementary element in the health work process that does not dispense with other approaches, such as clinical assessment, in the sense of the extended clinic, to identify other physical alterations that result from leprosy. Thus, the scales should be used to broaden and not limit the work of the professional. At this point, it should be noted that all the basic health units in the municipality studied have manuals that guide the use of the scales.

In this way, it can be understood that the proposed instruments are intended to mediate health work, without interfering in the worker's autonomy, since they do not define the entire work process in advance, but they can be a qualifying instrument in the work of nurses of great importance for planning health care for people affected by leprosy.

Finally, it should be emphasised that in addition to the studies that will validate the Ministry of Health's SALSA and Social Participation scales, the study in question reveals that these scales are easy to apply and effective in determining the physical and social condition of those affected by leprosy for subsequent planning of the necessary actions, and can be used in nursing work with patients after discharge or in leprosy treatment.

CHAPTER 6

BIBLIOGRAPHICAL REFERENCES

ALVES.C.J.M. et al. Evaluation of the degree of disability of patients diagnosed with leprosy in a Dermatology Service in the State of São Paulo. **Revista da Sociedade Brasileira de Medicina Tropical** . v 43, n. 4, p. 460-461, jul-ago. 2010.

AQUINO, D. M. C. et al . Profile of leprosy patients in a hyperendemic area in the Amazon region of Maranhão, Brazil. **Rev. Soc. Bras. Med. Trop**, v. 36, p. 57-64, jan. Uberaba, 2003.

ARANTES.C.K. Evaluation of health services in relation to early diagnosis of leprosy.**Epidemiol. Serv. Saúde**. v.19, n.2, p.155-164, abr-jun. Brasília, 2010.

ARAÚJO.M.G. **Hansen's disease in Brazil.** Rev. Soc. Bras. Med. Trop. v. 36, n.3, p. 373-382. Uberaba. May-June 2003.

BAIALARDI K.S. O estigma da hanseníase: relato de experiência em grupo com pessoas portadoras. **Hansen Int**. v.32, n.1, p. 27-31. Rio Grande do Sul, 2007.

BARBOSA, J. C. et al.Post-discharge leprosy in Ceará: limitation of functional activity, risk awareness and social participation. **Rev. bras. enferm.** v.61, p. 727-733, nov. Brasília, 2008.

BONITA, R. **Basic epidemiology**. 2.ed. - São Paulo. 2010, Santos.

BRAZIL. Ministry of Health. Health Policy Secretariat. Department of Primary Care. **Guide to leprosy control**. Brasilia: Ministry of Health, 2002.

_____. Ministry of Health. Health Surveillance Secretariat. **Epidemiological surveillance guide / Ministry of Health, Health Surveillance Secretariat.** 6. ed. Brasília: Ministry of Health, 2005.

_____. Ministry of Health. Health Surveillance Secretariat. Department of Epidemiological Surveillance. **Manual de prevenção de incapacidades / Ministério da saúde, Secretaria de Vigilância em Saúde, Departamento de Vigilância Epidemiológica.** 3 ed., rev. and expanded -Brasilia: Ministry of Health, 2008a.

_____. Ministry of Health. **Manual de Condutas para tratamento de úlceras em hanseníase e diabetes**. 2 ed. Brasília: Ministry of Health, 2008b.

_____. Ministry of Health. Health Surveillance Secretariat. Epidemiological Surveillance Department.**Management report of the General Coordination of the National Leprosy Control Programme - CGPNCH : January 2009 to December 2010 / Ministry of Health, Health Surveillance Secretariat, Epidemiological Surveillance Department.** Brasília : Ministry of Health, 2011.

_____. Ministry of Health Secretariat for Health Surveillance Department of Epidemiological Surveillance National Leprosy Elimination Programme. **National Plan for the Elimination of Leprosy at municipal level** 20062010. Brasilia, 2006.

CUNHA M.D et al.Leprosy indicators and elimination strategies in an endemic municipality in the state of Rio de Janeiro, Brazil. **Cad. Saúde Pública**, v.23, n.5, p. 1187-1197, mai. Rio de Janeiro, 2007.

COUTO. M.T et al. Men in primary health care: discussing (in)visibility from a gender perspective. **Interface - Comunic., Saude, Educ.**, v.14, n.33, p.257-70, apr.jun. 2010.

DIAS, R. C.; PEDRAZZANI, E. S. Políticas públicas na Hanseníase: contribuição na redução da exclusão social. **Rev. bras. Enferm**. v. 61, n. especial, p. 753- 756, nov. Brasília, 2008 .

DINIZ L.M et.al . Retrospective study of leprosy relapse in the state of Espírito Santo. **Journal of the Brazilian Society of Tropical Medicine**. v. 42, n. 4, p. 420-424. 2009.

DUARTE.C.T.M; AYRES.A.J; SIMONETTI.P.J. Nursing consultation: a strategy for caring for leprosy patients in primary care. **Texto Contexto Enferm**, v.18, n.1, p. 100-107. Florianópolis, 2009.

FAVARATO. M.E.C.S.Qualidade de Vida em Portadores de Doença Arterial Coronária: Comparação entre Genders. **Rev Assoc Med Bras.** v. 52, n. 4, p. 236-41, 2006.

FERREIRA .A.C. et al. Knowledge and practical behaviour of primary health care professionals regarding leprosy in the state of Tocantins, Brazil. **Cad . Saúde Colet.** v.17, n.1, p 39-50. Rio de Janeiro, 2009.

FIGUEIREDO, N. M. **Práticas de Enfermagem Ensinando A Cuidar em Saúde Pública.** Ed. São Caetano do Sul : Diffusão Paulista de Enfermagem, 2005.

GIL, C.A. **Como elaborar projetos de pesquisa**. 4 ed. São Paulo: Atlas, 2006. 175p.

GIROTI .S.K; NUNES.E.F.P.A ; RAMOS.M.R.L. As práticas das enfermeiras de uma unidade de saúde da família de Londrina, e a relação com as atribuições do exercício profissional. **Semana: Ciências Biológicas e da Saúde,** v. 29, n.1, p. 9-26, jan./jun. Londrina, 2008.

GOMES. D.C.C et al . Clinical and epidemiological profile of patients diagnosed with leprosy in a reference centre in the northeast of Brazil. **An Bras Dermatol.** v. 80, n. 3, p 283-288. 2005.

GUSMÃO, A.P.B., ANTUNES, M.J.M. Having leprosy and working in nursing: a story of struggle and overcoming. **Rev. Bras. Enferm.** v.62, n.6, p. 820-824, dez. Brasília, 2009.

HELENE, L. M. F; SALUM, M. J. L. The social reproduction of leprosy: a study of the profile of leprosy patients in the city of São Paulo. **Cad. Saúde Pública**. v. 18, n.1, p. 101-113, jan-feb. Rio de Janeiro, 2002.

IKEHARA E. et al.Salsa Scale and World Health Organisation Disability Grades: assessment of activity limitation and disability in leprosy **ACTA FISIATR.** v. 17, n.4, p. 169-174, nov. 2010.

IMBIRIBA. E.B, et al . Epidemiological profile of leprosy in children under fifteen years of age, Manaus (AM), 1998-2005. **Rev. Saúde Pública**. v. 42, n.6, p. 1021-1026. 2008.

JÚNIOR. A.F.R; VIEIRA.M.A; CALDEIRA.A.P. **Aspectos Epidemiológicos Da Hanseníase no Município De Montes Claros.** 2012. Available at http://www.mce.unimontes.br/index.php/enfermagem/mce/paper/view/47/31. Accessed on : 03 August 2012.

LANA F.C.F et al.Detection of leprosy and the Human Development Index of municipalities in Minas Gerais, Brazil. **Rev. Eletr.Enf**. v.11, n.3, p. 539-44, 2009.

LUNA. I.T et al. Adherence to leprosy treatment: difficulties inherent to patients**. Rev Bras Enferm**, v. 63, n. 6, p. 983-90, nov-dez. Brasília, 2010.

MACKERT. C.C.O. **Estudo de Base Popacional de Fatores Epidemiológicos de Risco em Hanseníase.** 96 p. Dissertation (Master's Degree in Health Sciences, area of concentration Medicine). Pontifical Catholic University of Paraná. Curitiba, 2008.

MARTINS. V; CAPONI. S. **Leprosy, exclusion and prejudice: life stories of women in Santa Catarina.** Ciênc. saúde coletiva**.** v.15, n.1, p. 1047-1054., jun. Rio de Janeiro, 2010.

MATTOS, D.M.; FORNAZARI, S.K. Leprosy in Brazil: representations and practices of power. **Cadernos de Ética e Filosofia Política** v.6, p. 45-57, 2005.

MATUMOTO.S; MISHIMA.M.S; PINTO.C.I. Collective Health: a challenge for nursing. **Cad. Saúde Pública.** v.17, n. 1, p.233-241, feb. Rio de Janeiro, 2001.

MARTELLI, C.M et al. Brazilian endemics and epidemics, challenges and prospects for scientific research: leprosy. **Rev. Bras. Epidemiol.** v. 5, n.3, p. 273-282. São Paulo, 2002.

MELAO.S et *al.* Epidemiological profile of leprosy patients in the extreme south of Santa Catarina, from 2001 to 2007. **Rev. Soc. Bras. Med. Trop**. v.44, n.1, p. 79-84. 2011.

MENDONÇA, A.V. et al . Immunology of leprosy. **An. Bras. Dermatol.** v.83, n.4, p. 343-350, aug. Rio de Janeiro, 2008.

MINUZZO.A.D. **The male leprosy patient: social representation, family social network, experience and body image.** 140 p. Dissertation (Master's in Well-being Policies in Perspective: Evolution, Concepts and Actors) University of Évora, 2008.

MIRANZI.C.S.S; PEREIRA.M.H.L; NUNES.A.A. Epidemiological profile of leprosy in a Brazilian municipality, from 2000 to 2006. **Rev. Soc. Bras. Med. Trop**. v.43, n.1, p .62-67, feb. Uberaba, 2010.

MOREIRA, T.M.A. et al. Leprosy in primary health care: effectiveness of training for health professionals in the State of Rio de Janeiro, Brazil. **Hansen. Int**. v.27, n.2, p. 70-76, 2002.

NUNES.J.M; OLIVEIRA, E. N; VIEIRA, N. F. Cunha. Leprosy: knowledge and changes in the lives of those affected. **Ciênc. saúde coletiva**, v.16, n.1, p. 1311-1318. Rio de Janeiro, 2011.

OLIVEIRA. M. H.P; ROMANELLI.G. The effects of leprosy on men and women: a gender study. **Cad. Saúde Públ.**, v. 14, n.1, p. 51-60, jan- mar, Rio de Janeiro, 1998.

WHO. World Health Organisation. **Operational Guidelines for the Implementation of the Global Strategy for Further Reducing the Leprosy Burden and Sustaining Leprosy Control Activities, SEA/GLP/2006.2** World Health Organisation South-East Asia Regional Office New Delhi, 2006.

___. World Health Organisation. **Enhanced global strategy for further reducing the leprosy burden: plan period: 2011-2015 / Pan American Health Organisation**. Brasilia : World Health Organisation, 2010.

World Health Organisation. **International Classification of Functioning, Disability and Health.** São Paulo: EDUSP; 2003.

PEREIRA,S. M.V. et al .Leprosy evaluation: nursing students' experience report. **Rev. Bras. Enferm.** v.61, n.especial, p. 774-780, nov Brasília, 2008.

SANTOS.R.N. Sistema Único De Saúde - 2010: Espaço Para Uma Virada. **The World of Health**, v. 34, n. 1, p. 8-19. São Paulo, 2010.

SCHOLZE.A.S et al.Strategic situational planning for leprosy control in the context of the psf: Experience from balneário Camboriú - SC. **Revista APS**, v.9, n.1, p. 39-44, jun. 2006.

SOBRINHO, R. A S; MATHIAS R.A. Perspectives for eliminating leprosy as a public health problem in the state of Paraná, Brazil . **Cad. Saúde Pública**. v.24, n.2, p. 303-314, 2008.

SOBRINHO, R.A et al. Evaluation of the degree of disability in leprosy: a strategy for sensitising and training the nursing team. **Rev. Latino-Am.** v.15, n.6, nov/dec. Ribeirão Preto, 2007.

PONTES. F. Increase in cases highlights the importance of rapid diagnosis. **Diário de Guarapuava**, Guarapuava, 16 and 17 January 2010, nº 2766, Regional Edition, p. 08 -11.

CHAPTER 7

APPENDIX 01: INFORMED CONSENT FORM

Dear participant

I would like to invite you to take part in the research entitled **"Applicability of the SALSA and Social Participation Scales as** nursing care **tools** for post-discharge and **leprosy** treatment patients**", which is part of the final course work for the** Nursing **course** at the Midwestern State University. The aim of the research is to assess the degree of functional activity limitation, risk awareness and social participation of post-discharge and leprosy treatment patients. For this, your participation is very important and will take place as follows: you will answer two questionnaires with multiple choice questions. We would like to inform you that you may have some doubts while answering the questionnaire, which will be explained by the interviewer. We would like to make it clear that your participation is completely voluntary and that you will not receive any payment for the research, nor will you incur any research costs, and that you may: refuse to participate, or even withdraw at any time without any harm to you. We also inform you that the information will only be used for this research and for scientific publication, and will be treated with the utmost anonymity and confidentiality, i.e. your name will not be mentioned at any time and all your data will remain confidential. The researcher is fully responsible for any damage resulting from the research. If you have any further questions or require further clarification, you can contact the researcher responsible for this project, whose contact telephone number is below. This form must be completed in two identical copies, one of which, duly completed and signed, will be given to you.

I, ____, declare that I have been duly informed and agree to participate VOLUNTARILY in the research coordinated by Prof. Ms Carine Teles Sangaleti Miyahara

____ Date:__________ _____ //2012

Participant's signature

Researcher's signature:____

Signature of supervisor:____

Any questions regarding the research can be answered by contacting the researcher below:

Jaqueline Fornari (42)99601048

Carine Sangaleti (42)36298134 (Contact from 2 to 6 pm at the Nursing Department of Unicentro).

ANNEX 01 : SALSA SCALE

ESCALA SALSA

Nome: ______________________ Idade: ______ Sexo: ______

Prontuário: ____________ Entrevistador: ______________________ Data: ___/___/___

	Domínio	**Escala SALSA** *Screening of Activity Limitation & Safety Awareness* (Triagem de Limitação de Atividade e Consciência de Risco) Marque uma resposta em cada linha	Se SIM, o quanto isso é fácil para você?			Se NÃO, por que não?		
			Fácil	Um pouco difícil	Muito difícil	Eu não preciso fazer isso	Eu fisicamente não consigo	Eu não faço por medo do risco
1.		Voce consegue enxergar (o suficiente para realizar suas atividades diarias)?	1	2	3		4	
2.	Mobilidade (pé)	Voce se senta ou agacha no chao?	1	2	3	0	4	4
3.		Voce anda descalço? i.e., a maior parte do tempo	1	2	3	0	4	④
4.		Voce anda sobre chao irregular?	1	2	3	0	4	④
5.		Voce anda distancias mais longas? i.e., mais que 30 minutos	1	2	3	0	4	④
6.	Autocuidado	Voce lava seu corpo todo? (usando sabao, esponja, jarra; de pe ou sentado)	1	2	3	0	4	4
7.		Voce corta as unhas das maos ou dos pes? e.g., usando tesoura ou cortador	1	2	3	0	4	④
8.		Voce segura um copo/tigela com conteudo quente? e.g., bebida, comida	1	2	3	0	4	4
9.	Trabalho (mão)	Voce trabalha com ferramentas? i.e., ferramentas que voce segura com as maos para ajudar a trabalhar	1	2	3	0	4	④
10.		Voce carrega objetos ou sacolas pesadas? e.g., com pras, comida, agua, lenha	1	2	3	0	4	④
11.		Voce levanta objetos acima de sua cabeça? e.g., para colocar em uma prateleira, em cima de sua cabeça, para estender roupa para secar	1	2	3	0	4	④
12.		Voce cozinha? i.e., preparar comida quente ou fria	1	2	3	0	4	④
13.		Voce despeja/serve liquidos quentes?	1	2	3	0	4	④
14.		Voce abre/fecha garrafas com tampa de rosca? e.g. oleo, agua	1	2	3	0	4	4
15.		Voce abre vidros com tampa de rosca? e.g., maionese	1	2	3	0	4	④
16.	Destreza (mão)	Voce mexe/manipula objetos pequenos? e.g., moedas, pregos, parafusos pequenos, graos, sementes	1	2	3	0	4	4
17.		Voce usa botoes? e.g., botoes em roupas, bolsas	1	2	3	0	4	4
18.		Voce coloca linha na agulha? i.e., passa a linha pelo olho da agulha	1	2	3	0	4	④
19.		Voce apanha pedaços de papel, mexe com papel/coloca papel em ordem?	1	2	3	0	4	4
20.		Voce apanha coisas do chao?	1	2	3	0	4	4
		Escores parciais	(S1)	(S2)	(S3)	(S4)	(S5)	(S6)
		Escore SALSA (*some todos os escores parciais*)	(S1 + S2 + S3 + S4 + S5 + S6)					
		Escore de consciencia de risco (*conte o numero de ④'s marcados em cada coluna*)						

ANNEX 02: SOCIAL PARTICIPATION SCALE

Escala de participação

Nome: ______________________ **Idade:**____ **Sexo:** ______

Prontuário: __________ **Entrevistador:** ____________________ **Data:** ___/___/___

Número	Escala de Participação	Não especificado, não respondeu	Sim	Às vezes	Não	Irrelevante, eu não quero, eu não preciso	Não é problema	Pequeno	Médio	Grande	PONTUAÇÃO
			0				1	2	3	5	
1	Você tem a mesma oportunidade que seus pares para encontrar trabalho?		0								
	[Se às vezes, não ou irrelevante] até que ponto isso representa um problema para você?						1	2	3	5	
2	Você trabalha tanto quanto seus pares (mesmo número de horas, tipo de trabalho, etc.)?		0								
	[Se às vezes, não ou irrelevante] até que ponto isso representa um problema para você?						1	2	3	5	
3	Você contribui economicamente com a sua casa de maneira semelhante à de seus pares?		0								
	[Se às vezes, não ou irrelevante] até que ponto isso representa um problema para você?						1	2	3	5	
4	Você viaja para fora de sua cidade com tanta freqüência quanto seus pares (exceto para tratamento), p. ex., feiras, encontros, festas?		0								
	[Se às vezes, não ou irrelevante] até que ponto isso representa um problema para você?						1	2	3	5	
5	Você ajuda outras pessoas (p. ex., vizinhos, amigos ou parentes)?		0								
	[Se às vezes, não ou irrelevante] até que ponto isso representa um problema para você?						1	2	3	5	
6	Você participa de atividades recreativas/sociais com a mesma freqüência que seus pares (p. ex., esportes, conversas, reuniões)?		0								
	[Se às vezes, não ou irrelevante] até que ponto isso representa um problema para você?						1	2	3	5	
7	Você é tão ativo socialmente quanto seus pares (p. ex., em atividades religiosas/comunitárias)?		0								
	[Se às vezes, não ou irrelevante] até que ponto isso representa um problema para você?						1	2	3	5	

Número	Escala de Participação	Não especificado, não respondeu	Sim	Às vezes	Não	Irrelevante, ou não queria/não preciso	Não é problema	Pequeno	Médio	Grande	PONTUAÇÃO
			0				1	2	3	5	
8	Você visita outras pessoas na comunidade com a mesma freqüência que seus pares?		0								
	[Se às vezes, não ou irrelevante] até que ponto isso representa um problema para você?						1	2	3	5	
9	Você se sente à vontade quando encontra pessoas novas?		0								
	[Se às vezes, não ou irrelevante] até que ponto isso representa um problema para você?						1	2	3	5	
10	Você recebe o mesmo respeito na comunidade quanto seus pares?		0								
	[Se às vezes, não ou irrelevante] até que ponto isso representa um problema para você?						1	2	3	5	
11	Você se locomove dentro e fora de casa e pela vizinhança/cidade do mesmo jeito que os seus pares?		0								
	[Se às vezes, não ou irrelevante] até que ponto isso representa um problema para você?						1	2	3	5	
12	Em sua cidade, você freqüenta todos os locais públicos (incluindo escolas, lojas, escritórios, mercados, bares e restaurantes)?		0								
	[Se às vezes, não ou irrelevante] até que ponto isso representa um problema para você?						1	2	3	5	
13	Você tem a mesma oportunidade de se cuidar tão bem quanto seus pares (aparência, nutrição, saúde)?		0								
	[Se às vezes, não ou irrelevante] até que ponto isso representa um problema para você?						1	2	3	5	
14	Em sua casa, você faz o serviço de casa?		0								
	[Se às vezes, não ou irrelevante] até que ponto isso representa um problema para você?						1	2	3	5	

Número	Escala de Participação	Não especificado, não respondeu	Sim	Às vezes	Não	Irrelevante, eu não quero, eu não preciso	Não é problema	Pequeno	Médio	Grande	PONTUAÇÃO
			0				1	2	3	5	
15	Nas discussões familiares, sua opinião é importante?		0								
	[Se às vezes, não ou irrelevante] até que ponto isso representa um problema para você?						1	2	3	5	
16	Na sua casa, você come junto com as outras pessoas, inclusive dividindo os mesmos utensílios, etc.?		0								
	[Se às vezes, não ou irrelevante] até que ponto isso representa um problema para você?						1	2	3	5	
17	Você participa tão ativamente quanto seus pares das festas e rituais religiosos (p. ex., casamentos, batizados, velórios, etc.)?		0								
	[Se às vezes, não ou irrelevante] até que ponto isso representa um problema para você?						1	2	3	5	
18	Você se sente confiante para tentar aprender coisas novas?		0								
	[Se às vezes, não ou irrelevante] até que ponto isso representa um problema para você?						1	2	3	5	

TOTAL

Comentário: ____

____

Graus de restrição de participação

Sem restrição significativa	Leve restrição	Restrição moderada	Restrição grave	Restrição extrema
0 – 12	13 – 22	23 – 32	33 – 52	53 – 90

ANNEX 03- APPROVAL SHEET FROM THE RESEARCH ETHICS COMMITTEE

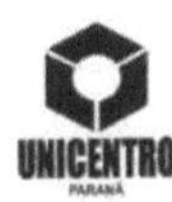

Universidade Estadual do Centro-Oeste

Reconhecida pelo Decreto Estadual nº 3.444, de 8 de agosto de 1997

COMITÊ DE ÉTICA EM PESQUISA - COMEP/UNICENTRO/G

Ofício nº 054/2012 - COMEP/UNICENTRO/G

Guarapuava, 27 de Março de 2012.

Senhora Professora,

1. Comunicamos que seu projeto de pesquisa intitulado: "Aplicabilidade das escalas SALSA e participação social domo instrumento do cuidado de enfermagem aos pacientes pós-alta e tratamento da hanseníase" folha de rosto nº 469666 parecer 259/2011 foi analisado e considerado **APROVADO** pelo Comitê de Ética em Pesquisa de nossa Instituição em Reunião Ordinária do dia 06 de Março de 2012.

2. Em atendimento ao Ofício Circular 017/2011 CONEP/CNS/MS informamos que é ***obrigatória a rubrica em todas as páginas do TCLE*** pelo sujeito de pesquisa ou seu responsável e pelos pesquisadores. As referidas assinaturas deverão ser apostas no fim de cada página.

3. Em atendimento à Resolução 196/96 do CNS, deverá ser encaminhado ao COMEP o relatório final da pesquisa e a publicação de seus resultados, para acompanhamento do mesmo.

4. Observamos ainda que se mantenha a devida atenção aos Relatórios Parciais e Finais na seguinte ordem:

- Os ***Relatórios Parciais*** deverão ser encaminhados ao COMEP assim que tenha **transcorrido um ano da pesquisa**.
- Os ***Relatórios Finais*** deverão ser encaminhados ao COMEP em até **30 dias após a conclusão da pesquisa.**

5. **Qualquer alteração na pesquisa** que foi aprovada, como por exemplo, números de sujeitos, local, período, etc. deverá ser necessariamente enviada uma carta justificativa para a análise do COMEP.

Pesquisadora: Carine Teles Sangaleti Miyahara

Atenciosamente,

Prof. Sueli Godoi
Coordenadora do COMEP/UNICENTRO/G
Port. Nº 2.053/2010 – GR/UNICENTRO

À Senhora
Prof. Carine Teles Sangaleti Miyahara
Departamento de Enfermagem - DENF/G
UNICENTRO

Home Page: http://www.unicentro.br

Campus Santa Cruz: Rua Salvatore Renna – Padre Salvador, 875 – Cx. Postal 3010 – Fone: (42) 3621-1000 – FAX: (42) 3621-1090 – CEP 85.015-430 – GUARAPUAVA – PR
Campus CEDETEG: Rua Simeão Camargo Varela de Sá, 03 – Fone/FAX: (42) 3629-8100 – CEP 85.040-080 – GUARAPUAVA – PR
Campus de Irati: PR 153 – Km 07 – Riozinho – Cx. Postal, 21 – Fone: (42) 3421-3000 – FAX: (42) 3421-3067 – CEP 84.500-000 – IRATI – PR

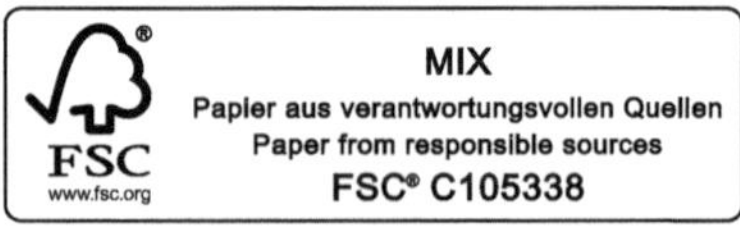

Printed by Books on Demand GmbH, Norderstedt / Germany